Welcome to the
Forsythe Cancer Care Center

Welcome to the Forsythe Cancer Care Center

Copyright © 2017, By James W. Forsythe, M.D., H.M.D.

All Rights Reserved, including the right of reproduction

in whole or in part in any form

Forsythe, James W. M.D., H.M.D.

1. Health 2. Homeopathy 3. Natural Remedies

ISBN -13:978-1546333418

Dedication

To all my past, current and future patients.

Discover Our Clinic's Vastly Superior Survival Rate

The five-year survival rate of advanced Stage IV cancer patients treated at my clinic, the Forsythe Cancer Care Center, is nearly 31 times better than the national average.

On a nationwide basis only a dismal 2.1 percent of all such patients survive after being treated by mainstream oncologists who deliver high-dose standard chemo.

By comparison, results at the Forsythe Cancer Care Center, also called Century Wellness Clinic, reflect a seven-year survival rate of more than 64 percent among such patients that I had treated at the time of this book's publication.

To put this into clear perspective, think of the situation this way: only two out of 100 advanced-stage cancer patients survive when treated by conventional cancer doctors. In sharp contrast, at least 68 out of every 100 similar people survive when I treat them. There are several reasons:

Unique tests: My clinic offers chemosensitivity genomic tests that determine which types of chemo will most effectively treat a specific individual, while also identifying which drugs, hormones and natural supplements work best for the patient.

Effective process: Before treatment begins, I meet with each patient to develop an effective treatment process based largely on results of the chemosensitivity tests.

Natural treatments: My clinic uses effective and safe natural treatments that refrain from damaging the body, while killing cancer and fortifying their natural immunity. These are unlike dangerous drugs used by mainstream oncologists who often administer harmful synthetic substances that destroy the patient's health and may lead to death. The treatment process involves insulin potentiated therapy or "IPT," where patients receive the two best drugs determined for them individually; this is done along with small amounts of chemotherapy at from 10 percent to 15 percent of standard doses, with insulin added.

Cancer obliterated: In most cases my unique treatments generate a 90-plus-percent kill rate of the cancers within such patients. This often enables the patients' immune systems to assume and to successfully carry out the job of completing our fight against the disease, leading to remission. The natural ability of my patients to kill off all remaining cancer increases significantly when I administer superior, effective immune-boosting natural substances.

The 64-percent cancer survival rate generated by the Forsythe Cancer Care Center reflects patients who will remain alive five years after treatment. Some survivors at that point may have at least some cancer; among many of these individuals the disease is considered "manageable." Most doctors generally refer to such patients as "cured," particularly individuals who remain in remission after five years.

Consider Me Unique

My treatments sharply boost the possibility of a cure, thanks to the fact that the chemosensitivity tests specify which drugs would work best, and which would be ineffective for each specific patient.

As noted in my newsletters for patients, thanks to the chemosensitivity tests made possible by genomics research, "no other oncologist in the United States can offer this kind of information to his or her patients. What conventional oncologists offer only is what has been the best results of the latest clinical study."

Those reports, which have nothing to do with chemosensitivity tests fail to generate 85-percent accuracy. In fact, many studies embraced by mainstream oncologists are only 30 percent to 50 percent successful.

Results show that conventional chemotherapy treatments administered by mainstream oncologists would never help one half to two thirds of Stage IV cancer patients.

Sadly, these patients are merely being poisoned when given chemotherapy, which does nothing to eliminate cancer--while intensifying their suffering.

Consider Me A Maverick Doctor

Before initially visiting my clinic, many patients soon realize that I'm one of just a handful of working "integrative medical oncologists" worldwide.

This means that I'm fully licensed to practice medicine as a mainstream certified medical oncologist, while simultaneously working as a board-certified Homeopathic physician using natural treatments.

"I essentially use what some people call 'the best of both medical worlds."I sometimes tell patients. "If I'm giving you the wrong drug, I'm killing you. But that's what traditional oncologists are doing every day."

My unique Forsythe Cancer Care Center, also called Century Wellness Clinic, located in Reno, Nevada, in the western United States, also fights cancer with harmless and effective natural substances. We do this without the excessive use of the poisonous, dangerous and expensive drugs such as high-dose chemo administered by mainstream oncologists.

Instead, depending on each patient's specific needs and results of the person's chemosensitivity tests, I develop individualized treatment regimens. These often include extremely limited regimens of low-dose chemo along with various natural remedies.

Sadly, mainstream oncologists are forced by the standard medical industry's required protocol to administer deadly regimens of high-dose chemo to all advanced Stage IV cancer patients--with no exceptions.

From the view of many mainstream doctors, I'm threatening to "overturn the proverbial apple cart."

Under such a scenario, would the resulting "public outcry" generate an ideal situation where frustrated patients worldwide and vote-hungry politicians insist that every mainstream oncologist order chemosensitivity tests for all cancer patients?

Patients Yearn for Effective Natural Remedies

Every week streams of patients from around the world travel to the Forsythe Cancer Care Center for treatment of cancer or other ailments.

Every week out-of-state license plates are seen in my clinic's parking lot, after patients drive from as far away as Maine, Florida, Alaska, Canada and Mexico.

This influx of visitors provides a consistent and significant boost to the Reno-area economy, generating thousands of hotel room occupancy rates per year, with average patient stays at least three to four weeks.

A noticeable portion of these patients from almost every continent. courageously visit my clinic, after being told by mainstream oncologists elsewhere tell patients to "get their affairs in order."

"Never take the word of any doctor who would tell you something like that," I say to patients. "Every patient needs to remain hopeful for as long as possible."

Genetics Research Makes this Possible

Much of the Forsythe Cancer Care Center's success in effectively treating cancer patients has been made possible by genomics research, along with my previously mentioned natural remedies.

These technological advances stem from studies inspired by the Human Genome Project, when scientists mapped out the entire human genome from 1990 to 2003.

Findings made possible by genomic research since then have enabled scientists to develop the amazing chemosensitivity tests. I consider this as an essential, vital and necessary tool for cancer doctors when developing effective individual treatment regimens. Yet keep in mind that as previously mentioned, mainstream oncologists insist on ignoring these techniques.

So, as you might imagine, I've been called a "maverick doctor," largely due to my unwillingness to follow the proverbial dictates of allopathic physicians.

You see, I refrain from "following the proverbial pack" of mainstream doctors. Instead, I choose to essentially stand in my own field while proudly enabling my patients to benefit from effective new genomic technologies that other doctors ignore.

Patients Benefit From Choices

My Stage IV cancer patients at the Forsythe Cancer Care Center are given a choice regarding their own treatment regimens.

This serves as a sharp contrast from the process offered by mainstream oncologists; those physicians refuse to enable patients to make such decisions.

At my clinic, patients who wish to go conventional at least know about the best drugs for them. At that point, they then have the right answer. We also offer low-dose (10%-15%) insulin-potentiated chemotherapy over a three-week period.

We also send all patients home with the appropriate supplements deemed highly effective for their individual cancers, renewing these products on an as-needed monthly basis. A re-evaluation at three to four months is always required.

Chemosensitivity Testing Works Wonders

Every year, tens of thousands or perhaps millions of cancer patients in the United States fail to receive genomics-generated cancer chemosensitivity tests that could save their lives.

In countless instances such procedures could prevent certain patients from receiving poisonous chemo that never would help them. When that happens high-dose chemo ravages their bodies. This invariably leads to extremely painful, horrendous and lingering death. Their bodies literally waste away.

"On a widespread social scale, this is a tragedy seemingly beyond belief," I tell patients who inquire about the issue. "The sad fact is that most mainstream oncologists either refuse to or fail to inform their patients that chemosensitivity tests exist."

From the standpoint of the vast majority of allopathic cancer doctors, everything essentially comes down to "guesswork" because of the dismal fact that they refrain from seeking such procedures.

Compounding the problem, as mentioned earlier, medical industry standards require mainstream oncologists to follow "protocol." These puzzling rules mandate that all patients with certain types of advanced-stage cancers always be given specific full-dose types of chemo drugs at a pre-designated, high-level; these are administered on pre-set schedules.

Disturbing Results Emerged

By my estimates, in the United States every day nationwide more than 1,300 cancer patients needlessly die such deaths--the equivalent of several jumbo jets crashing into the ocean.

The amount of human suffering is immeasurable on a grand scale.

Yet why do mainstream doctors refuse to recommend such tests? Does mainstream medicine's close ties with Big Pharma--the giant multi-billion-dollar pharmaceutical industry--have anything to do with such the disturbing behavior of these physicians on a grand scale?

While no one can accurately give an irrefutable answer to these critical questions, at least something is clear--patients need to be proactive.

Demand Such Tests

Any person suffering from cancer, particularly advanced Stage IV levels of the disease, should demand the option of taking such tests before any chemo begins. Here are the steps such patients should take:

Access: Before treatment begins, tell the doctor that you want a "cancer chemosensitivity test."

Options: Inquire about what options are available from the doctor for receiving such tests.

History: Ask if the doctor has ever given patients access to such procedures.

Red Flags: Be on the lookout for a "red-flag warning" if the physician refuses to offer these tests.

Avoid Conventional Oncologists

When I tell my clinic's cancer patients about this, they immediately start avoiding mainstream oncologists--often telling many people that they know to do the same.

I have been issuing such warnings for many years.

In fact, as I noted in my clinic's October 2010 newsletter, "gene testing has the answers" for cancer patients seeking to benefit from cutting-edge technology.

From my view now in my fifth decade of practicing cancer medicine, the development of such tests emerged as "the biggest C-change in all my years of practice with more than 200,000 patient visits."

Patients Appreciate Access

At the Forsythe Cancer Care Center, the advent of cancer chemosensitivity testing has made a major difference in the lives of our patients' success levels and improved overall survival rates. These statistics became evident in our present, ongoing seven-year, 1,200-patient study.

Drawing whole blood at my clinic, cancer chemosensitivity tests are relatively simple, easy and productive procedures. Upon their initial visits to the Forsythe Cancer Care Center, some people with cancer are what Homeopaths call "virginal treatment patients."

The designation signifies that those individuals have not yet been treated for their cancers, and therefore have never been subjected to potentially dangerous or deadly treatments such as multiple drugs, radiation, or even major surgery.

For the most part upon their initial visits to the Forsythe

Cancer Care Center, these patients know that their disease is advancing, and their prognosis is guarded. They know their time factors are limited and they want real answers, along with effective non-toxic treatments.

Avoid the Guessing Game

Most of them highly educated and extremely inquisitive, these patients want to avoid getting ensnared in the type of "guessing game" used by mainstream oncologists.

With equal importance, as I clearly stated in my 2010 newsletter, these patients "don't want an oncologist that picks out drugs and throws them against a wall to see if any stick in terms of their own cancer response rates."

A highly trained and experienced member of my professional staff begins the chemosensitivity testing process by taking a patient's whole blood--a very simple and easy procedure. The blood is then handled very carefully, while undergoing stringent packaging and shipping requirements; samples remain good for up to 96 hours prior the time when the Greek laboratory analyzes the sample.

My personnel always draw the blood on the first part of the week, ensuring that the sample gets to its destination in a safe, preserved and fresh manner.

Upon arrival at the testing laboratory, scientists and lab technicians subject the blood to high-tech tests. At last count, my clinic estimated that at least three labs worldwide provide this service-- one in Germany, one in Greece and one in South Korea.

We Fine-Tuned Efforts

Following several years of testing, at the Forsythe Cancer Care Center we found that the Greek Test offers the most important information in terms of the number of chemotherapy agents and supplements that are tested along with the greatest accuracy.

To its credit, the Greek company, RGCC, Research Genetic Cancer Centre, tests at least 18 families of chemotherapy agents and 38 families of supplements.

Once RGCC receives the blood, the testing process takes from 10 days to two weeks for completion of the analysis. To do this, the lab's technicians and scientists sample and harvest the cancer cells-- which are then cultured in vitro for gene analysis.

These specific characteristics within the patient's genes are then compared in relationship with how--if at all--the various chemotherapy agents interact with these markers. This way lab technicians determine which of the specific drugs and 38 supplements work best, if any. In "hormone-driven" cancers the test identifies the best agents for hormonal control.

Upon completing this thorough analysis the Greek laboratory sends results to me. Then, after carefully reviewing this vital data, I construct a protocol involving a unique effective formula that marries the two most effective conventional drugs with all the best supplements. Once a patient agrees to pursue such a strategy, I often combine natural remedies and low-dose chemo to "work smart, rather than merely working hard." Small doses of insulin (5-10 units) are used to augment the low-dose chemotherapy.

Mainstream Oncologists
Destroy the Body

The vast majority of advanced Stage IV cancer patients who visit conventional clinics are merely being poisoned by chemo that fails to do anything to eliminate their cancer. High-dose chemo often causes:

Chemo-brain syndrome: Commonly called "post-chemotherapy cognitive impairment," this hampers or wrecks the patient's cognitive abilities. According to the "Journal of Clinical Oncology," from 20 percent to 30 percent of people who undergo chemotherapy experience at least some form of chemo-brain syndrome. These outcomes have been so disturbing that the Journal of the National Cancer Institute has designated the condition as a real, measurable side effect. Some cancer survivors complain of a degradation of their cognitive abilities, plus decreases in their fluency and memory.

Cardiac toxicities: Sometimes called "cardiotoxicity," this condition occurs when the heart muscle sustains damage and the organ's ejection fraction reduces. These adverse characteristics, in turn, weaken the heart--which fails to adequately pump. The blood circulates with less efficiency than the organ had previously managed to accomplish consistently prior to the chemotherapy treatments. This can be measured by testing the ejection fraction (EF), which should be above 55 percent.

Peripheral neuropathies: This dreaded condition occurs when the body's sensory nerves become damaged or diseased. The numerous adverse symptoms that vary among patients can include the impairment of organs or glands, and severe pain, plus a hampered ability of movement and a decrease or loss of sensation. A vast array of additional nerve-related damage sometimes occurs, depending on which portion of the body's nerves are effected.

Bone marrow suppression: Sometimes called "myelotoxicity," this adverse medical condition generates one or all of numerous highly adverse effects. Besides the potential loss of normal blood clotting, some patients experience severe infections that result from a decrease in the white cells responsible for providing immunity. Just as destructive, another condition called "anemia" can severely hamper the essential life-giving ability of red blood cells to carry oxygen.

Generalized rashes: Often lasting from five to 20 days, or perhaps much longer, this condition can generate bothersome itchiness, bumps, cracked or blistered skin, debilitating pain, and a variety of other adverse conditions such as secondary infections due to cracks or blisters.

Death: Conventional oncologists typically prefer to avoid discussing this topic at length with patients, but there is no escaping the fact that the needless or reckless over-use of chemotherapy often results in unnecessary death. Quite predictably many patients suffer from some or even all of the previously mentioned symptoms triggered by chemo, before dying from severe levels of these adverse side effects. Most allopathic cancer doctors refrain from admitting this disturbing fact--many of their patients are killed by the highly toxic and poisonous chemo, rather than succumbing to the cancer itself.

Better Choices Available

As a licensed oncologist I'm required by law and by industry protocol to give each Stage IV cancer patient the option of having conventional high-dose chemo "treatments"--instances where such a strategy would be required of standard oncologists.

The vast majority of people with advanced-stage cancer who visit my clinic freely choose to avoid high doses of dangerous drugs.

These patients usually follow my recommendation of a low-dose insulin potentiated chemo regimen, coupled with effective natural remedies--as determined by genetic testing.

For these individuals, my clinic administers low-dose fractionated insulin-potentiated regimens often referred to as "IPT." This technique "tricks the cancers" into opening up certain biological receptors. This happens due to a cancer's enhanced supply of insulin receptors. Amazingly, this is how PET scans work.

These attributes leave the cancer open to potentially effective attacks by apoptosis-producing natural Poly-MVA administered by my clinic's medical personnel. This tactic often works because cancers can manage to "die off."

As a result, the cancers often die or go into remission, robbing the disease of its ultimate goal of killing the patient.

Important Book Emerged

One of my many patients became so impressed with this process that she wrote a compelling book about her positive experience being treated at the Forsythe Cancer Care Center.

Las Vegas-based businesswoman Diana Warren chronicled her story in "Say No to Radiation and Conventional Chemo--Winning My Battle Against Stage II Breast Cancer."

Prior to visiting my office Warren had gone to numerous mainstream oncologists. All of those medical professionals had insisted that she endure high-dose chemo treatments and radiation therapy.

Brave, intelligent and charismatic, Warren refused to cave in to their dangerous medical procedures. Instead, she let common sense serve as her guide, while ignoring the reckless protocol of mainstream physicians.

Warren undertook an in-depth research regimen, eventually deciding to visit my Reno-based clinic 450 miles from Las Vegas. Then, at my urging, Warren decided to take the "Greek Test," the chemosensitivity analysis.

The test results arrived within several weeks. Right away I worked with Warren in developing her personalized treatment regimen. We used a combination of the medications and supplements that the analysis had identified as the most effective for her body and particular type of cancer.

Warren's unique and specialized low-dose chemo treatment regimen began within several weeks at the Forsythe Cancer Care Center. Her cancer went into remission soon afterward, and at the time of this book's publication she had remained in remission for more than four and a half years before sustaining a reversible relapse.

Numerous Positive Outcomes

Although I would never refer to myself in such glowing terms, numerous doctors and industry observers refer to me as a "virtual rock star within the medical industry."

Rooms filled with Homeopaths and their assistants often erupt into applause or give standing ovations as soon as I enter some medical industry conferences.

Always in high demand to attend such functions, I usually visit from six to 10 medical industry seminars yearly throughout the United States. You see, I continually learn more about fighting cancer while always developing effective, natural ways to fight the disease.

The positive focus on me and my clinic's techniques intensified when an intelligent and highly respected celebrity, Suzanne Somers, mentioned these critical details in worldwide media forums. Somers became so impressed that she described my clinic's cancer treatment procedures in her runaway 2010 bestseller, "Knockout: Interviews With Doctors Who are Curing Cancer--And How to Prevent Getting It in the First Place."

Huge percentages of my patients learn of the Forsythe Cancer Care Center via positive word-of-mouth from other people previously treated at my clinic. Streams of my patients first learn about me in Somers' book, or from the many books that I have written, or co-authored, or from publications where other writers praise my medical procedures.

Groundbreaking Doctor
Pushes the Proverbial Envelope

An internationally acclaimed Los Angeles physician and surgeon, Doctor Patrick Soon-Shiong, has generally been using the same overall type of genomic-related testing and cancer treatment that my Forsythe Cancer Care Center has been using with much success.

With an estimated personal worth of $11 billion, Soon-Shiong has been called "a genius, a showman, an innovator and a hipster," CBS News correspondent Doctor Sanjay Gupta, said in a "60 Minutes" program segment first aired on Dec. 7, 2014.

Like me, Soon-Shiong has had his advance-stage cancer treatment methodology come into question from some mainstream doctors. Those physicians insist that more time is needed to determine if such genomic testing and low-dose treatments are effective and worthy of being recommended.

Yet as if echoing statements that I have made for several years, Soon-Shiong told Gupta that patients suffering from advance-stage cancer lack the luxury of time needed to wait for extensive testing and federal approval of new treatments.

"I'm incredibly encouraged to say that we are on the path," Soon-Shiong told "60 Minutes." "And the technology to do these things is not just hypothetical."

Soon-Shiong insists that scientists are learning to unmask cancer's molecular secrets, thanks largely to advances in DNA technology, coupled with a high-speed genome sequencing machine that he developed.

Similar to a process that I implemented at my clinic, the billionaire doctor prefers to have his advance-stage cancer patients undergo genomic testing. Like me, he strives to determine which specific drugs have the greatest probability of effectively killing the cancer of each patient.

Another similarity to my clinic's general protocol emerges from the fact that Soon-Shiong prefers administering low-dose chemo treatments.

Similar Overall Techniques Lead to Success

In yet another significant similarity, Soon-Shiong insists that many people have a mistaken belief that cancer cells merely "grow." Instead, because of a mysterious and still-misunderstood genetic mutation, the worst cancers essentially have the inability to die.

In our separate, unaffiliated medical practices while still employing similar overall strategies, Soon-Shiong's clinic and mine share a mutual professional and highly focused obsession with using genomic technology to determine the characteristics of cancer's strange mutation.

Ultimately, this often results in an improved long-term survival rate, always starting with a thorough analysis of each individual patient's genomic structure and specific type of cancer.

In best-case scenarios, these advances in cancer diagnosis and treatment ultimately lead to instances where the disease becomes categorized as completely gone or when cancer evolves into a "chronic health conditions" rather than fatal.

"Overall, these advancements are clicking into gear at a far greater pace than many people realize," I sometimes tell patients. "The old way of treating cancer patients with high-dose chemo should quickly emerge as 'a thing of the past,' replaced by a much more effective era."

Forsythe Cancer Care Center Leads the Way

Almost every day the whole world seems to be banging on my clinic's door, eager and desperate to benefit from substantial advances in genomic technology.

Yet amazingly only an infinitesimal fraction of the 7 billion living people worldwide knows that my clinic uses these amazing anti-cancer techniques.

My office doors are always open weekdays, except on a handful of U.S. holidays and during the brief span from Christmas through New Year's Day.

As you might very well imagine, my office phones are continually "ringing off the hook" while people ask for appointments.

Many patients tell me that they're pleased and delighted upon discovering that my staff is eager to answer any questions that they might have.

Demand Continues to Intensify

The patient load at the Forsythe Cancer Care Center continues on a steady increase. Every step of the way we strive to make the process as stress-free and easy as possible for each person eager for an examination and treatment.

I have already stated the following in the first chapter, but I need to re-emphasize the details here because the important facts are essential to all my patients:

Many people vising for the first time admit they're impressed by the fact that nearly two-thirds of my Stage IV cancer patients remain alive and in remission from the disease--seven years after their initial treatments at the Forsythe Cancer Care Center.

Remember, this means that six out of every 10 worst-stage cancer patients that I treat remain alive, most relatively healthy and capable of enjoying life to the fullest.

By contrast, according to numerous nationwide medical reports, only two out of every 100 Stage IV cancer patients survive when treated by mainstream oncologists at only five years.

So, knowing these details, who would you choose--the doctors required to administer high-dose poison in all such cases, or me, an expert at administering an effective combination of low-dose chemo, natural remedies and healthy supplements?

Take These Important Steps

To help optimize results and make their excursions as stress-free as possible, all first-time patients visiting the Forsythe Cancer Care Center can:

Call: 775-827-0707, or toll free 877-789-0707; tell the receptionist your health situation, so that we can start the process of potentially making a reservation.

Records: Upon making a reservation, you must bring copies of your records from your current doctor, or send us that information before arriving. This information should include any and all available reports regarding oncology, pathology, surgery, chemotherapy, X-rays, scans, laboratory tests, narrative summaries, and a list of all medications and supplements.

Frailty: Like all doctors, we generally are unable to treat patients who have become "extremely frail;" under this condition the person's body mass and weight have dropped to precipitously low levels--while muscles have severely wasted.

Prior Treatments: Preferably before their first visit to the Forsythe Cancer Care Center, patients should avoid being treated elsewhere by mainstream oncologists. The high-dose chemo and radiation administered by those doctors seriously weakens and damages the body--thereby decreasing the potential effectiveness of subsequent treatments. Homeopaths refer to people with cancer who refrain from chemo and radiation prior to visiting doctors of natural medicine as "virginal treatment patients." Although we prefer treating "virginal patients," in many instances my clinic accepts people with cancer who already have been treated by conventional oncologists. In order to be accepted, such candidates must communicate with a member of my staff before a decision is made.

Travel & Accommodations: New and returning patients make their own arrangements for travel and lodging. The Reno area has numerous high-quality hotels and restaurants at mid-range and high-end prices. Car rentals via Reno-Tahoe International Airport are available for those who travel by air, and shuttle services are provided by most major hotel-casinos in the region.

Location: The Forsythe Cancer Care Center, also called Century Wellness Clinic, is at 521 Hammill Lane in South Reno, an ideal site just one block from on-ramps and off-ramps to U.S. Interstate 580--one of the region's two primary highways. A north-south arterial, I-580 provides easy access to the airport, all of the region's primary hotels, and the region's primary east-west highway, U.S. Interstate 80. Travel time to or from the airport and the clinic is about 10 minutes.

Activities: During "free" time when not undergoing medical examinations or treatments, patients, their relatives or friends have a vast array of options for fun, relaxing, energizing or restful activities. The high-desert region surrounding Reno, which is at 4,500 feet above sea level, has hundreds of miles of hiking trails providing panoramic views. The city is just a one-hour drive from Lake Tahoe, an ideal summer playground. Nestled in the Sierra at 6,200 feet above sea level, as North America's largest alpine lake, Tahoe has easy access to dozens of ski resorts popular during winter. Just as enticing, the historic Comstock Lode mining town of Virginia City, where the legendary writer Mark Twain began his journalism career for the "Territorial Enterprise" in the 1860s, is just a 30-minute drive southeast of Reno. Virginia City has numerous popular attractions including museums, and historic saloons such as the the world famous Bucket of Blood saloon.

Expected stays: Patients visiting for initial examinations and chemosensitivity testing usually stay from several days to one week.

Those undergoing treatment regimens of low-dose chemo, effective natural remedies and supplements usually stay from two to three weeks. Subsequent visits for standard examinations are usually recommended for patients who have undergone treatments, so that I can monitor each person's progress in beating cancer. Follow-up visits for examinations usually are arranged in three- or six-month, or one-year intervals; these spans hinge on the type of cancer a patient had, the current suspected severity of the disease; and whether the cancer has gone into--or seems to progressing into--remission.

Additional treatment: Some patients occasionally require or request follow-up treatment regimens if their cancer remains active following the initial round.

Various ailments: The Forsythe Cancer Care Center treats patients suffering from many types of ailments, particularly cancer. We treat all types of the disease in any bodily area and at every level of severity; besides advanced Stage IV cancer, the clinic treats patients suffering from less severe levels including Stage II and Stage III. Patients need to know that unless effectively treated all types of cancer can worsen to the dreaded Stage IV; the worst-stage cancers invariably lead to death unless successfully treated. In addition, many patients learn prior to their initial visits to the Forsythe Cancer Care Center that mainstream oncologists strive to administer poisonous and deadly high-dose chemo to patients suffering from the less severe Stage II or Stage III levels of the disease--not just Stage IV.

Critical Patient Choices

Keep in mind that as previously stated, throughout every phase of each patient's examinations and treatment I give the patient the option of making critical choices.

This marks a sharp contrast from the style of mainstream

oncologists, who essentially say without using such specific words: "It's my way, or the highway."

I give each patient the option of receiving natural remedies that are proven highly effective, always with the patient's physical and mental well-being in mind.

In doing so, I'm essentially following the philosophy of Doctor Benjamin Rush, a signer of the Declaration of Independence and the personal physician of U.S. President George Washington.

"Unless we put medical freedom into the Constitution, the time will come when medicine will organize into an undercover dictatorship," said Rush, a founding father of the United States who died in 1813 at age 67. "To restrict the art of healing to one class of men and deny equal privileges to others will cause a Bastille of medical science.

"All such laws are un-American and despotic, and have no place in a republic. The Constitution of this republic should make a special privilege for medical freedom."

To the detriment of all types of patients, no such provisions were included in the USA's founding documents. Since then mainstream doctors have run roughshod over patients' rights; these physicians have used their political allies to implement and control federal agencies that require or sanction the use of ineffective, costly, and poisonous deadly drugs.

Whole Body and Soul

Effectively treating patients can only happen when addressing the whole body, the mind and what I sometimes call the person's "positive spirit or soul."

Unlike mainstream oncologists who poison the entire body in an effort "to fix an isolated cancer," I incorporate a whole-body strategy using mostly natural remedies.

Besides administering low-dose chemo with natural remedies, personnel at my clinic also help address numerous issues in order to improve each patient's overall health. Among these critical health-enhancing tactics that mainstream oncologists ignore are:

Balance: We show each patient how to achieve a balanced lifestyle using an ideal combination of rest, exercise, sleep, nutrition and activities suited for emotional harmony.

Detoxify: Clean the body of foreign or unnatural substances that are likely to damage overall health, while sometimes also sometimes triggering cancer.

Diet: The common saying that "you are what you eat" remains true, sometimes leading to cancer due to unhealthy diets. So, we teach patients about good nutrition.

Empower: As previously stated, we give each patient choices about treatment, recovery and strategies to achieve or to maintain optimal health.

Information: We teach patients the critical details that they must know to detect, prevent and control cancer.

Sugar: We teach each patient that common sugars, particular when ingested in high amounts, are a leading cause of cancer--which "love and thrives" on this substance.

Supplements: Use the supplements identified by chemosensitivity testing as the most helpful for a specific cancer patient; these products contain vitamins, minerals and various herbs. They serve as the backbone for good overall physical, mental and spiritual health.

Target Specific Cancers

I have developed unique, individualized strategies to effectively battle each form of cancer.

This is unlike mainstream oncologists who--as previously stated--use an ill-advised and ineffective "one-size-fits-all" approach to almost every form of the disease.

By analyzing an individual's chemosensitivity test, physical examination and medical records, I'm able to marry the best natural remedies in combination with low-dose chemo, along with supplements identified as the most effective for the person.

Doctors classify each form of cancer based on the bodily area where the disease started. Compounding the challenge, each type of cancer has a unique growth rate, pattern of spreading and response to specific treatments.

Many physicians and particularly Homeopaths have deemed me as perhaps the world's premiere expert at developing and matching the ideal and most effective treatment for each type of cancer.

Chemosensitivity tests are particularly helpful because each person has a unique, one-of-a-kind genomic structure unlike any other person.

Risk Factors Play a Role

Intense and continuous worldwide genomic research has been identifying and confirming what many physicians have suspected for a long time.

Genomic research has confirmed that some individuals have a greater likelihood than the general population of developing specific types of cancer.

For instance, women from some families have a far greater chance of developing breast cancer than most females throughout the general population.

At least some good news has emerged. Scientists have confirmed that the inherited probability of cancer is less prevalent than previously thought.

As a result, some researchers and medical facilities have informally categorized most cancer causes as instances where the individual is a victim of "bad luck."

Many severe risk factors sharply increase the probability of getting cancer. Besides smoking or chewing tobacco, these include exposure to chemicals, ultraviolet light, free radicals in foods, red or processed meats, sugar, air pollution and many more.

In addition, each specific risk factor increases a person's chances of getting certain cancers. For instance, smoking or chewing tobacco sharply increases a person's risk of developing cancers of the lung, tongue, mouth, larynx, and other organs. Scientists blame most skin cancers on excessive exposure to the sun or suntanning parlors.

Most tumors are benign or lacking cancer; such tumors are usually non-threatening, except in rare exceptions.

In all instances of cancer, a person's chances of "being cured" increase drastically the sooner the disease is discovered and treated; cancers that are allowed to grow and spread over extended periods without being treated sharply increase the chances of developing into deadly advanced Stage IV levels of the disease.

My War in Fighting Cancer

In the fight against cancer, patients at the Forsythe Cancer Care Center might think of me as a proverbial five-star general or a commander-in-chief.

Under my continual command the clinic's staff administers at least 17 strategies, many that I have personally designed to destroy cancer. With added importance, some of these strategies strive to put each patient on a pathway toward optimal overall health.

Besides the unique chemosensitivity testing of whole blood, one of these key techniques briefly mentioned earlier involves the low-dose fractionated regimens sometimes called "IPT."

As previously stated, when using a unique system that I personally developed, the process strives to "trick" or "fool" the disease into opening certain receptors within the cancer's cells. This happens in part because cancers desperately crave energy-producing sugar and thrive in low-oxygen and acidic tissues.

I work to ensure that this natural process opens biological receptors. When this happens the cancer is left wide-open to horrific attacks, while the rest of the body remains unharmed and safe.

The typical weaponry that I employ here involves a natural substance, the harmless and effective Poly-MVA expertly administered by my staff. This is usually done on alternate days with low-dose fractionated chemotherapy, levels much smaller and far less harmful to the body than chemo typically administered by mainstream oncologists.

Napoleonic Battles Against Cancer

Although despotic, often cruel and heartless, the famed French Emperor and my clinic treats people with other health issues that compromise or weaken immunity.

Biological Response Modifiers: Besides the immune enhancement technique listed immediately above, we also employ "biological response modifiers" that are sometimes called "BRMs." Remember that as mentioned earlier, the effective strategies that I employ typically strive to kill at least 90 percent of a patient's cancer, and from that point the person's immune system plays a critical role in fighting and successfully killing the remainder of the disease. Similar to substances naturally produced by the body and often created by scientists in laboratories, BRMs super-charge the body's natural response to infection and to cancer. This "immunotherapy" treatment process enhances the body's immune systems, particularly natural defenses against cancer. Also, because my clinic serves patients with ailments other than cancer, we sometimes use BRMs to affectively address such adverse conditions as rheumatoid arthritis. Although comprised of natural substances, the administering of BRMs on extremely rare occasion generates adverse symptoms such as diarrhea, nausea, vomiting and loss of appetite. Thus, BRMs should only be taken in a professional medical environment that monitors patients.

Bio-Oxidative Therapy: A super-powerful tool among natural healing methods, the natural process called "bio-oxidative therapy" serves as a stong anti-oxidant and cancer killer. Unlike humans and all mammals, cancer gets its oxygen from the fermentation process, rather than breathing from the environment. At my recommendation and upon patient approval, I use bio-oxidative therapy to surround cancer cells with oxygen. This high-oxygen environment can significantly decrease the disease's ability to grow and to divide. Meantime, this therapy typically stimulates receptors in white blood cells, thus boosting the immune system and fortifying the body's natural strength and effectiveness in attacking cancer. Perhaps just as impressive, this therapy increases the body's natural production of interferon, interleukin-2 and tumor necrosis factor--all factors that sharply boost the body's natural cancer fighting processes. Meantime, bio-oxidative therapy also often improves the health of patients who have been ill, thanks to the ability of this process to increase oxygen tension in bodily tissues.

Lifestyle guidance: Clinic staff members often teach or suggest ways for an individual patient to enjoy life to the fullest extent possible. Such positive behavioral changes often make the person feel better both physically and emotionally, thereby decreasing the likelihood that a cancer will worsen or return. When giving this advice, my personnel consider numerous simultaneous factors including the person's type and severity of cancer, level of remission, overall health, and all other ailments currently experienced by the individual.

Professional referrals: As a highly experienced doctor with extensive medical industry contacts throughout Northern Nevada and worldwide, I sometimes refer patients who need additional services to other medical professionals ranging from surgeons to radiation therapists.

Second opinions: After initially receiving the diagnosis of physicians elsewhere, some people visit the Forsythe Cancer Care Center to seek a "second opinion" from me and other doctors on my staff. Sometimes we reach similar conclusions, although in numerous instances either I or my personnel generate findings that differ from what the patient had been told elsewhere.

Coping skills: Forsythe Cancer Care Center offers individual and group counseling, unlike the vast majority of mainstream oncologists and cancer treatment facilities nationwide. At my clinic, skilled advisers highly knowledgeable in medicine and optimal lifestyles teach patients or their families how to cope and excel in key issues. Patients and their families learn optimal ways to administer effective healthcare, plus suggested methods on handling daily lifestyle tasks or personal responsibilities.

Napoléon Bonaparte of the early 19th Century remains world-famous for his dastardly war tactics of suddenly attacking enemies using extreme unconventional tactics.

At least within the realm of battling cancer, many of my patients think of me as using "Napoleonic battle plans against the disease within the practices of both oncology and Homeopathy."

Highly detailed books could be separately written and published about each of my most popular and effective cancer-fighting strategies. Besides chemosensitivity tests, IPT, and low-dose fractionated chemotherapy, here is a brief summary of some of the most effective methods frequently used at the Forsythe Cancer Care Center:

Healthful water: Because healthful, pure water can boost energy while ridding the body of harmful and potentially cancerous impurities, we provide patients with access to "alkaline H2O pH therapy." The water is at an optimal alkaline level, the opposite from the harmful acidic range. This strategy serves an important role because cancer thrives within an acidic environment; the pH levels of cancer patients are typically far more acidic than alkaline.

Nutritional guidance: What a person chooses to eat plays a critical role in either generating or preventing cancer. Many of these "poor" and "good" choices hinge on whether a particular food is within the healthful alkaline or unhealthy acidic ranges. We show patients meal plans developed for their unique personal situations. These details can be found in my book, the "Forsythe Anti-Cancer Diet;" it's available in paper or e-reader form via all major bookstores and online eBook venues.

Individualized nutrition: Besides the advice on diet briefly mentioned above, we develop cancer-fighting and cancer-preventing regimens that include specific foods, vitamins, and herbs. As I often tell patients, natural substances such as these generally are far more preferable than unnatural or synthetic drugs typically administered by mainstream oncologists. Besides helping to boost overall health, such products serve as just one of the many ways that we help give the body a fighting, natural chance against cancer.

Immune Enhancement: Cancer typically compromises or wrecks the body's immune system, often robbing the person of energy and the ability to fight the disease. To counteract this detrimental condition, we administer a high-dose Vitamin-C immune booster that patients receive intravenously as a standard procedure. Often loaded with vital additional vitamins and supplements, these immune-enhancing sessions often sharply increase the body's natural ability to battle certain ailments--particularly cancer.

Patients Deserve Priority Status

At the Forsythe Cancer Care Center, every patient gets "priority status;" they all deserve and receive respect without being ignored or told, "Do this and do that. Take this poison, because you have no other choice."

The doctors and personnel at my facility strongly embrace this highly coveted mission statement. We strive to show each patient that the clinic truly cares, while effectively working in an effort to achieve the best possible results.

Blessed with a keen knowledge of the art and science of medicine, I continually draw upon all treatment modalities ranging from the most advanced conventional therapies to mainstream medicine. All along, I also incorporate the most effective remedies of Homeopathic medicine, primarily natural therapies ignored by mainstream oncologists.

Using these medical systems as a solid foundation for giving all patients the best possible care, I have developed four options uniquely designed to fulfill their desires:

One: Fractionated conventional chemotherapy alone

Two: Fractional low-dose chemotherapy, plus Homeopathic treatments including Insulin Potentiated Therapy (IPT)

Three: Complimentary Homeopathic and/or naturopathic modalities alone

Four: Best supportive therapy

Based on my intensive studies, I have discovered that superior results occur when using combination treatments of: fractionated (low-dose) chemotherapy; Homeopathic intravenous remedies; and immune-stimulating supplements including organic herbs.

Along with my staff throughout the course of treating thousands of patients, I have developed intense studies on: Paw-Paw, a naturally grown substance deemed highly effective in cancer treatment; Poly-MVA, a uniquely formulated combination of minerals and amino acids designed to support cellular energy and promote overall good health, while also highly effective for treating cancer; the Forsythe Immune Protocol, a highly effective immune-enhancing process that I personally developed to significantly boost positive results in the treatment of my cancer patients; and a combination of the Forsythe Immune Protocol, CST and IPT.

A "Bill of Rights" for Patients

Determined to counteract the "dogmatic rules" imposed by mainstream oncologists who refuse to allow patients to make vital choices regarding their own health, I have developed an essential "Bill of Rights" that all people with cancer can embrace. Among some of the most important proclamations:

Positive attitude: Each patient has a right to refrain from becoming afraid or discouraged, always cognizant that at various times in recent years medical literature has chronicled cures for all types of cancer.

Alternative path: Patients have a right to chose a unique, extremely rare integrative medical oncologist such as me because I'm highly skilled at treating their entire bodies with harmless and effective natural remedies--plus drugs when necessary.

High-dose chemo: Patients have a right to refuse extensive high-dose chemo regimens that mainstream oncologists insist on administering. When and if such a refusal is made, the patient should have a right to seek out the services of an extremely rare integrative medical oncologist such as me--capable of administering effective natural remedies.

Remain skeptical: Patients have a right to "keep an open mind about issues," while also remaining skeptical when reading or hearing about the supposed results of various clinical studies--particularly instances where two or more drugs are used.

Show spunk: Each patient has a right to peacefully "stand his or her own ground" as a self-preservation measure. Such instances might involve politely leaving an oncologist's office when the doctor mentions "hospice care" or "getting your affairs in order." Such statements indicate that the physician has given up on you; all patients have a right to embrace an attitude that: "I will never give up on myself."

Food choices: Patients have a right and a responsibility to themselves to adopt good eating habits, following the advice of their Homeopaths, physicians and dietitians.

Avoid unnecessary tests: Patients have a right to refuse over-testing, particularly procedures that involve radiation; radiological scans that target various areas of the body's overall immune system are particularly dangerous. Such procedures endanger overall health, increasing the likelihood that immune defenses will fail to work at optimal levels. These include bone scans, CAT scans, and PET scans.

Alternative medicines: Patients have a right to know about, to use and to benefit from effective natural remedies that mainstream oncologists refuse to mention or to use. Of particular importances are beneficial supplements that often emerge as extremely helpful and essential in fighting cancer; supplements also eliminate carcinogens and toxins from the body.

Beware of media: Patients have a right and a responsibility to themselves to remain wary of advertisements or promotions that strive to fool them. For instance, some cancer centers claim to have the latest "pinpointed radiology procedures."

Refuse certain surgeries: Particularly among those with advanced Stage IV cancer, patients have a right to avoid a doctor's insistence that they undergo aggressive surgical procedures. These include second-look operations and devastating head-and-neck surgeries requiring tracheotomy and/or gastric feeding tubes.

Limit drugs: Patients have a right to limit the amount of drugs that they take. Whenever possible a patient should be able to take the smallest number of drugs, administered at the lowest-possible doses needed to fight their cancer. This strategy can minimize or prevent the destruction of the person's vital immune system.

Patients Praise Me

I receive heart-felt, compelling and emotional letters or emails each week from all over the world, sent by patients extremely grateful for their improved health.

"I'm so grateful to remain alive," is a phrase signifying a common theme. "I'm eternally grateful for the new lease on life that you have given me."

Some of my now-healthy former patients retell their stories, recounting the fact that they had previously been told elsewhere that: "You are going to die."

Imagine being informed that you are definitely going to be killed within a certain limited number of weeks or months, only to subsequently learn after finally being treated by me that you are going to live.

While glad to receive these messages, I refrain from dwelling on them--partly due to the need to continually concentrate on my job of "saving" as many people as possible.

Of course, not all of my patients survive. Yet as previously stated, the five-year survival rate of my advanced Stage IV cancer patients is far greater than the national average. Remember, according to my clinic's current study involving 1,200 patients, only two out of every 100 Stage IV cancer patients treated by mainstream oncologists survive, while at least 64 of such people that I treat remain alive at seven years.

Essential Details

As previously mentioned, even following my success in treating cancer patients, I never can, have or will issue any guarantee that any patient will be cured or experience a significant improvement in his or her overall medical condition.

With this clearly understood, readers should remain fully cognizant of the fact that the details that I have provided in this book are strictly for educational and informational purposes only.

In addition, you should refrain from considering any or all statements that I have made here as medical advice--specifically because at this point we can assume that you are not yet a patient of mine.

I only make specific diagnosis and issue recommendations individually to each of my patients after conducting a thorough physical examination and reviewing medical records.

With these "disclaimer" factors clearly understood, my clinic welcomes inquiries from potential patients. Also, prospective patients should know that the Forsythe Cancer Care Center, also known as the Century Wellness Clinic, is an out-patient facility without overnight accommodations.

About the Author

James W. Forsythe, M.D., H.M.D., has long been considered one of the most respected physicians in the United States, particularly for his treatment of cancer and the legal use of human growth hormone. In the mid-1960s, Dr. Forsythe graduated with honors from the University California at Berkeley and earned his Medical Degree from University of California, San Francisco, before spending two years residency in Pathology at Tripler Army Hospital, Honolulu. After a tour of duty in Vietnam, he returned to San Francisco and completed an internal medicine residency and an oncology fellowship. He is also a world-renowned speaker and author. A retired full Colonel in the Nevada Army National Guard, he has co-authored, been mentioned in and/or written chapters in bestsellers and other popular books. To name a few: "Stoned ~ The Truth About Medical Marijuana and Hemp Oil;" "The Human Genome Playbook for Disrupting Cancer;" "An Alternative Medicine Definitive Guide for Cancer;" "Knockout, Interviews with Doctors who are Curing Cancer" Suzanne Somers' number one bestseller; "Victory Over Cancer ~ Using the Best of East and West Medicines;" "The Ultimate Guide To Natural Health, Quick Reference A-Z Directory of Natural Remedies for Diseases and Ailments;" "Anti-Aging Cures;" "The Healing Power of Sleep;" and "Compassionate Oncology ~ What Conventional Cancer Specialists Don't Want You To Know;" and "Obaminable Care," "Complete Pain," "Natural Pain Killers," and "Your Secret to the Fountain of Youth ~ What They Don't Want You to Know About HGH Human Growth Hormone," "Take Control of Your Cancer," "Understanding and Surviving Obamacare," "About Death from a Cancer Doctor's Perspective," "Dr. Forsythe's Whey Protein Anti-Aging Formula," and the "Emergency Radiation Medical Handbook," and "Maverick M.D." His newest book is currently in produciton, "Essential Oils in the Treatment of Cancer."

Contact Information

Forsythe Cancer Care Center,
also known as Century Wellness Clinic

521 Hammill Lane

Reno, NV, 89511

(775) 827-0707

RenoWellnessDr@Yahoo.com

DrForsythe.com

Made in the USA
San Bernardino, CA
08 March 2018